LOSE WEIGHT FAST: 101 WAYS TO LOSE UP TO 10 POUNDS IN 7 DAYS

JEFF ANDERSON

INTRODUCTION

Hello and welcome! Thank you for downloading Lose Weight Fast: 101 Ways to Lose up to 10 Pounds in 7 Days!

It is common knowledge that we as Humans will always seek to answer our questions and solve our mysteries. Since the dawn of our existence, we have always had a massive question: *How to successfully lose weight with little to no effort?*

The Weight-Loss industry is one that moves billions of dollars annually, as men and women of all ages seek all kinds of methods (new or old) to get rid of those extra pounds that make them uncomfortable. It is perhaps a gift or maybe a curse that we always look for perfection in our appearance and lifestyle.

In the following book, we will not delve into the mysterious corridors of miracle medicines; or attempt to teach you complicated fitness routines. *No!* Our goal here is to help you become a fit, healthy human being; by using our simple, bite-sized tips that will not only give you great space to choose your desired methods of shedding those annoying extra kilos...but also have fun in discovering new and incredible ways of becoming a fitter person!

The best part of the book you are reading is not only that these tips have been certified by experts and are proven and efficient ways to lose weight, but also that they are *guaranteed* to help you lose up to 10 pounds in 1 week! That's ten in one! You *definitely* read that right.

So get ready, you'll find tips and suggestions that range from diets to types of exercises, new lifestyles or just simple things you can do to help yourself lose weight!

With all of that said...Good luck, and remember, nothing changes if YOU don't change!

TABLE OF CONTENTS

24. Don't punish yourself with unrealistic goals!

25. Coffee is allowed, but...there's always a but!

26. Do you like swimming? You will now!

27. Drink LOTS of Water!

28. Avoid stress, just stay away from it!

29. If you have to break the rules, break them gracefully!

30. Consider Yoga, it's the weight-loss ally!

31. Fit apps, something our parents didn't have!

32. Avocado is the new Meat!

33. The couch isn't your final destination!

34. Kids are angels, and pregnancy weight-gain is temporary!

35. As any great adventure, everything must be Gradual!

36. Patient Eating is Key!

37. Don't skip breakfast!

38. Take it easy on weekends and days off!

39. Smile, and above all, laugh!

40. Stay positive and ignore any dumb Comments!

41. Rearrange your Environment!

42. Find a hobby you can do at Home!

43. Follow a Schedule!

44. Look for like-minded people to share your Experiences with!

45. Hate that belly? Burn it down with sit ups and a healthy diet!

46. Dine healthy, Dine early!

47. Prioritize on making your own Food!

48. Climb like your life depends on it!

49. Remember jumping rope as a kid? Now do it for Real!

50. Waiting rooms? More like fat-gaining rooms!

51. No more selective parking!

52. Unsure of the balance on your plate? Check out the colors!

53. Make sure you choose the right Meat to Eat!

54. Jog as often as you can!

55. Find the Fiber in your Life!

56. Not a sporty person? Try other fat-burning Activities!

57. So you can't even step outside? You look Great! Come on!

58. Be sure you know Exactly what you want!

59. No more excuses; this isn't a favor, it's a commitment!

60. The Experts know best, don't be afraid to Ask!

61. Discover your true Ideal Weight!

62. No more Oil or Butter: Get a non-stick pan!

63. Don't put your health at risk for an extra day of Gym or Jogging!

64. Also, don't risk worsening an injury for a few burned Calories!

65. Kids keeping you from exercising? Not if you play with them!

66. READ-THE-LABELS!

67. Not helping much at home? Get Involved!

68. Enjoy your video games? Why not try out some Fitness on them?

69. Safety first: Don't go out without the right kit for your workout!

70. Less sleep, more exercise? No, more sleep, more exercise!

71. Your bed isn't just for sleep though...*wink*

72. Protein Shakes aren't just for Muscle-heads!

73. Best time of day for Weight Loss? In the Morning!

74. If it's something you can't live with...Don't live without it!

75. Be careful with what you're Told!

76. Also, don't believe in Miracle Fat Burners!

77. No pain, No Gain!

78. Exhaustion is a good sign!

79. It's a Myth that you need to be rich to Lose Weight!

80. Go out, even if it's alone!

81. Healthy Competition is just that: Healthy!

82. Shower instead of having a Bath!

83. Don't kill the Flavor!

84. The best moment to exercise might not actually be the Best!

85. Tired of Salads? Get some Soup!

86. Reap the Rewards!

87. Keep a record of what's good for you and what's Not!

88. Breathe in, Breathe out; Breathing before Eating!

89. Smaller Plates; Smaller Problems!

90. Going out somewhere? Don't expect the unknown, eat at home!

91. The Golden Rules!

92. Get your Heart beating and your Fat Burning with Cardio!

93. "But I want to lose weight, not get stronger!" Ugh!

94. If you can't manage today, you will tomorrow, or after!

95. Don't think of taking breaks!

96. Eat like you're Posh!

97. Chewing makes the difference!

98. Don't obsess; your Fun Adventure could turn into a Horror Story!

99. The Perfect Diet!

100. Pay Great Attention to these Tips!

101. Enjoy every Minute!

Final Notes

LOSE WEIGHT FAST: 101 WAYS TO LOSE UP TO 10 POUNDS IN 7 DAYS

Welcome back! As you were told in the Introduction, the following are tips that will help lead you through the otherwise tough process of shedding extra pounds. It is important to note that they aren't written or placed in any particular order or category.

Enjoy reading and applying them to your life, good luck!

DON'T STARVE YOURSELF!

One of the most common mistakes done mostly by young females is to stop eating altogether, starving themselves of valuable nourishment in order to lose weight — but our bodies don't work that way! *Yes*, you will lose fat, but eating only one meal a day will slow our metabolism down and weaken us (Our body will still take its necessary energy from other places, like muscles!). By the time you're done fasting, you'll be sick, tired and once you start eating again, you'll gain weight faster than you did before (That's where the metabolism part kicks in), so avoid this method of shedding fat!

Take your Dog out for a daily Walk!

Why not give your dog a treat at the local park by taking him or her for a run? Sometimes walking or running isn't very fun, but it can be, especially when you've got your furry companion chasing the ducks or pigeons. It will also benefit from your exercise, since it will get some as well. After a few weeks, the both of you might look *much* better and fitter than you did before you started! Remember to stretch, and try to be constant and punctual. Pets will get used to their walks, and won't like it if you get lazy!

GO WALKING WHEN YOU NEED TO THINK!

Does your job require you to apply many brainstorms, planning or imagination? What about simple accounting or keeping memory of inventories? I'm pretty sure that you must use your brain for at least *one* of the things at your job, or you wouldn't be needed (Lame joke)! Try to get up and walk around when you're thinking. It's one of the most useful ways of exercising when you're doing something else and you feel "busy". Perhaps the *only* way to exercise at work, unless you have a heavy physical job. In that case, keep it up!

FANCY TAKING A TAXI OR BUS FOR SHORT RIDES? NOT ANYMORE!

It is a common *bad* habit to find the quickest route to our destinations and just hop onto a taxi or bus to go somewhere close. *Don't!* Unless you're in an unsafe area, always try to walk, take the longest, safest route you have and you'll notice that it will become a habit. In fact, your wallet will also soon be grateful, since you'll be saving all of that pocket money you used to spend! PS: You'll also be helping keep the environment that little bit cleaner and less polluted!

ELEVATORS, ESCALATORS? NO! STAIRS, YES!

Remember how you used to go searching for the elevators and escalators in every mall and building you visited, even your apartment blocks? Well, those days are over. From now on, *always* and I cannot stress that 'always' enough, go for the stairs. You may have seen the irony of how people would rather wait in a line to get onto an elevator instead of climbing the stairs which are only a few feet away, well, don't be one of those people! You'll improve your fitness not only in weight, but in flexibility, endurance and other attributes.

GOT A GARDEN? DON'T YOU THINK IT DESERVES A LITTLE OF YOUR TOUCH?
Gardening. Something typically left to an employee or a relative who loves your front yard. Time to get dirty, I think! When you're free from work and chores, dedicate an hour to your garden, plant some trees or vegetables or flowers or...whatever! And tend to them when you can. This type of hard work is one of the most efficient at dropping weight, since you have to put quite some effort into it. You may not want to stop helping out your neighborhood gardener with the extra cash, and if that's the case, feel free to help him out. You'll be a nicer person for it as well!

DON'T SHOP WHEN YOU'RE HUNGRY!

While saying this out loud, it sounds kind of silly doesn't it? But it's not. If you use your own memory to recall the last time you went shopping, you'll remember that you probably bought some extra snacks, ice cream, chips or at least *some* kind of fatty food because you couldn't wait to go home and eat it. Yeah, don't smile; I *know* it was that way, because it happens with everyone. Try to have a decent meal before going shopping and take a list! That way you know what you're going to buy and can ensure that you won't make any unnecessary runs to the snacks aisle.

CHORES AREN'T BORING IF YOU DANCE!

Those dreaded dishes. The sticky kitchen floor. That untidy bedroom upstairs. You're probably rolling your eyes just imagining these phrases. What if I told you, that you could make cleaning *fun?* All you have to do is get to your PC, Cell phone or Sound System and put some music on! Make sure it's something you can dance, grab that broom or mop and you'll be finishing quicker than ever, as well as getting some exercise done at the same time! *Ah, if only you could do it in public, huh?*

DROP THE UNHEALTHY HABITS!

Yeah, I know. You've already tried to stop smoking and/or drinking several times to no avail. Even so, it's not helping you out; in fact it's damaging your precious body. Treat your body like a temple, you wouldn't throw poison into a sacred place would you? The worst problem arrives when you justify your bad habits by saying "Smoking/Drinking is what keeps my mind off eating," but that isn't an excuse. It's still hurting you, much more than fat is (in the long run). Seek to get rid of these habits, you're not helping anyone.

Nobody is to Blame!

Well, okay, Dad always brings chocolates from the store. And maybe your little brother always shares his candy with you. Hey, don't forget all those fast food commercials, or the fact that you can *never* resist going for a burger at night at the local diner. Still, that doesn't mean you have to lay the fault of those extra pounds on yourself or worse, on somebody else! I recommend you read up on *Body Composition.* Everyone's body composition is different, which is why two people with the same weight can have totally different bodies! Keep in mind that things like genetics, adaptation and other external factors come into account when it comes to our bodies. Just focus on getting rid of that fat, and being positive!

KEEP TRACK OF YOUR PROGRESS!

There's no point in starting something this big if you're not going to pay attention to the results! As soon as you can, get a scale and a mirror, and make sure to take note of anything you found that really helped, or on the contrary, hindered your objectives in shedding weight. Do this regularly (*Not obsessively*), at least twice a week, and you'll realize how well you're doing with yourself. It will make you want to keep going, and you'll be able to tell people how many pounds you've lost!

COOKING FOR ONE? MAKE SURE IT'S JUST FOR ONE, THEN!

A common mistake that is made when cooking is "More is better than less" which could normally be interpreted as acceptable, but *not* when you're trying to lose weight. When you cook more than you need, you'll typically end up eating a bigger portion than you intended. This means you'll be getting more food than you need or even want! Try to control and measure how much it is you're cooking, and don't go looking for more once you're done. Either that, or give the excess food to a nearby friend/family member, they'll love you for it!

KEEP YOUR HANDS OFF THAT DESSERT!

Now, do you *really* need to go for that Chocolate Fudge, or that Strawberry Cheesecake after that large meal (I'm sorry if I made you think of them)? Not really. Dessert can be the fattiest food you'll eat all day, and arrives into your stomach at the point where you're least likely to burn that fat, since you're already full up. Some experts recommend eating desserts *first*, but I'd got a step forward and recommend you to eliminate it from your diet altogether, unless you don't mind trading those chocolate bars for an apple, or some nuts (More on these later). If so, *go ahead!*

BAKE AND GRILL, DON'T FRY!

This is one for those out there who love their burgers, their meat, their chicken…There are other ways to eat it than fried. Some may sigh in dismay, but fried food is something you will need to slowly remove from your diet. It's not doing you any good at all. All of that oil and fat is going to do damage on your body in the future, too. I shouldn't have to tell you that health issues such as diabetes, kidney disease, heart attacks and **cancer** can be a result of the continued consumption of fried foods. Even our brain has a chance to function abnormally when consuming sunflower or flaxseed oils, among others.

TAKE SUPPLEMENTS FOR PERFECT BALANCE!

You've probably seen a family member carrying around their small pot of vitamins, and maybe you've wondered if you might need them yourself. Why yes, of course! Even if you're under the strictest and most efficient diet, and you're doing exercise 7 days a week, you'll need to strengthen your body in certain aspects that'll inevitably be missing. Be sure to take supplements, though a visit to the doctor might be necessary beforehand just to make sure.

EATING OUT CAN BE HEALTHY!

Yeah, believe it or not. While some experts will recommend to *stop* eating out, as social creatures, that's impossible. So let's set a realistic milestone. Let's trade the unhealthy fast food for the healthier meals. Find out more about vegetarian/vegan cuisine in your area, or healthy yogurt bars. Make sure you're still having fun with your friends while being healthy, since you can't give up one part of your life just because of another! Life is more than getting thinner, don't forget that!

TRY 'LIGHT' AND 'REDUCED FAT' VERSIONS OF YOUR FAVORITE FOOD!

Remember, being on a strict diet doesn't mean not eating anything delicious — you still can! Next time you buy your typical yogurt, butter, ice cream or chocolate spread, go for the Light version. Even so, be aware that you can't abuse these, because despite them having less calories than your typical version of the chosen product; some nutritionists and psychologists have noticed that people will eat *more* than usual when they know they're eating a less fatty version. They also contain more chemicals, to allow the product to possess equal amounts of flavor and color.

CHANGE YOUR PLATE'S COLOR!

"Just what the heck, is this a joke?" I can almost hear you ask. Well, no! According to experts, the color **blue** will make people eat less than when eating on red or yellow plates. Further studies proved that it wasn't necessarily the color, but the *contrast* between food and plate. Red food (such as tomato-based sauce) will disappear on a red plate, but not on a green one. Be aware of this, and serve food on contrasting plates!

GREEN TEA IS A MIRACLE BEVERAGE!

Seriously, I cannot stress this enough. Green Tea possesses so many benefits to your body, whether or not you want to lose weight. It's loaded with antioxidants, increases fat burning and metabolic rate, lowers the risk of cancer, kills off bacteria and keeps Type II Diabetes away, among other excellent and healthy things. Be sure to consume a cup or two daily, it will keep you young and healthy!

Keep those Sauces and Dressings off your food!

Remember, all of those additions you make to your meal are calories, and if they're all just a craving, then you *can* avoid them. For example, Mayonnaise (A main component of many dressings) is mostly fat and calories. Keep your salad dressings to vinegar, olive oil and salt. It will make an already healthy food, healthier! As for those special sauces, they require to be cooked, which means oil, which means fat. Self-explanatory, really.

LET YOUR FRIENDS KNOW THAT YOU'RE ON A MISSION TO LOSE WEIGHT...
I'm not telling you to be insistent and boring about it, but proudly announcing that you're on a diet and might not be able to go to fast food restaurants anymore, and will spend some of your leisure time at the gym or running on the beach is enough! That will make sure that they respect your diet and training, and who knows, perhaps there's even a chance that...

...AND YOU COULD ALSO GET THEM TO JOIN IN!

There's no harm in suggesting to your friends in a tactful manner that you guys and/or girls don't look like you used to, and since you've started to look for a change in your weight and appearance, they're welcome to join! At least one or two of them will consider it, and soon you'll be having more fun as you run, as well as eating healthier in company. Who knows, maybe they'll thank you in the end for helping them out!

GO NUTS EATING NUTS!

Well, that was just a catchy phrase for the tip, but you get my point. I previously mentioned eating Nuts was a positive thing for weight-loss seekers, and now it's time to explain. Nuts are packed with healthy fats, proteins, vitamins and minerals. Eating them will typically give you the feeling of being full, despite not having to eat much, and they can substitute any snack. The four best types are Almonds, Walnuts, Cashews (A personal favorite) and Pistachios. Go for raw versions of nuts, never the oily or fried kind.

DON'T PUNISH YOURSELF WITH UNREALISTIC GOALS!

Now, I know you'll set goals like looking like a supermodel within a couple of months; doing a *Liquid Diet* for weeks; or doing a lap around the city daily, but these things are frankly not going to happen, or at least you won't feel happy at doing them for longer than a few days. Don't hurt your ego and hope by setting unrealistic goals. Follow the tips in this book and any material you may find online or with experts, and you'll be fine! It's healthier and safer to lose weight gradually than to do it all in one shot, anyway.

COFFEE IS ALLOWED, BUT...THERE'S ALWAYS A BUT!

For those who just can't live without coffee, that's okay! You're allowed to have your morning cup of Joe. Now, however, you're going to need to switch cream and sugar for skimmed milk. You'll be shedding 105 calories off your normal intake in one shot, not bad for a single cup of coffee, huh?

DO YOU LIKE SWIMMING? YOU WILL NOW!

Swimming is called one of the fittest sports, since you work *all* of your muscles, top and bottom, and you'll develop an excellent body if you keep it up! Now, experts may recommend squash, ultimate Frisbee, tennis and other sports for weight loss...but how many of us actually have time for that? On the other hand, you can visit the local pool every evening or at least a couple of days a week and have some fun swimming across the pool or even *walking* across it! You'll exercise, lose body fat and have fun.

Drink LOTS of Water!

Water has *no* calories. Yes, you read that right. You can drink as much as you want, and not only will you feel full, but you won't gain any weight for doing so! Here's where it gets better: water also helps speed up your metabolism and ensures a better digestion, so you won't just look better with time, but *feel* better as well! In fact, drinking a cold glass or two of water before meals and after waking up should make sure your metabolism is working at top gear!

Avoid stress, just stay away from it!

Stress is a killer. Really, I'm not kidding you. Stress can lead to muscle pains, headaches, chronic illnesses and the common bad mood you'll be carrying all week long. But as if that wasn't bad enough, stress can make you gain weight. How? Well by making you eat, or by keeping you from exercising, or simply just ruining your self-esteem all around. All of these things will indirectly lead you to start gaining weight again. Just keep away from stress, try meditation, look up hobbies that can keep your mind occupied and try to share your load with family, friends and/or partner. Be happy!

IF YOU HAVE TO BREAK THE RULES, BREAK THEM GRACEFULLY!

What I want to say here is: Yeah, you're allowed the occasional chocolate bar or ice cream cone…But that doesn't mean that when you go for one, you're going all out and asking for doubles with toppings! Come on, now. The same rule applies for skipping your exercises. Don't turn a "day off" into a "lie all day on the couch day". That's just regression, and regression is *bad* for you while you're losing weight. Either pause or go forward, never backward!

CONSIDER YOGA, IT'S THE WEIGHT-LOSS ALLY!

Yoga isn't just a thing that rich CEO's do while they're not making millions or that old people love. It's an incredible practice that has many, many benefits to your body. You'll find that it can improve flexibility and muscle strength, as well as protect your bones and spine. What does it have to do with weight loss? Well, it lowers your blood sugar, eases digestive problems and you'll burn up to 350 calories in one hour of practicing it! That's more than you'll burn in one hour in a jogging/walking combination. Awesome!

Fit apps, something our parents didn't have!

I'm not going on an advertising mission here, but there are certainly many apps out there that can make life easier in our modern times. Try downloading one or two to your phone, like a calorie-counter, a workout log or a running app that keeps track of your daily distance. They'll help you make sure you're constantly keeping up your level, and will also ensure you know how much of a gradual increase you're making on your exercises (Because you'll have to get past the easy stuff once you've gotten used to it, and turn a 1 km run into a 5 km one and so on)!

AVOCADO IS THE NEW MEAT!

Yep, believe it or not, you can actually substitute meat for avocado in many meals (Not necessarily all, unless you're going vegan). They're rich in fiber and healthy fats, as well as vitamins and minerals. The Avocado isn't known as a superfood for no reason! You'll also be losing weight, because it's a healthier and equally tasty replacement for meat, with its soft but firm texture and pleasant flavor. Try it out, but don't eat the skin or seed!

THE COUCH ISN'T YOUR FINAL DESTINATION!

Remember that when you're watching TV, you can also stand up on commercial breaks and walk around. A sedentary lifestyle is a known cause for premature death (Sitting still for at least 5 hours a day is a great risk on its own, regardless of exercise). Obesity is just one of the many consequences of leading a sedentary lifestyle, so please, please, please! Avoid sitting on the couch or chair in front of your computer for many hours without even moving around. It might cost you later on life, as well as keeping you from losing those annoying pounds!

KIDS ARE ANGELS, AND PREGNANCY WEIGHT-GAIN IS TEMPORARY!

This tip is for the girls: There will probably come a time in your life when you receive the great news...you're having a *baby!* Once the congratulations have arrived and you're getting used to life as a Mother, you begin to notice something...you're getting chubbier by day. *Oh dear, what now?* Experts point out that the best condition to be in to get pregnant is when you're *not* overweight, but nevertheless...You should always try exercising and diets after having your child (or children) as well as breastfeeding them to lose those pounds of baby fat. Becoming a mother isn't the end of your beautiful body, don't give up!

As any great adventure, everything must be Gradual!

There are **big** mistakes you can make when trying to lose weight, but one of the **biggest** is expecting instant results, or instantly giving up your normal lifestyle in the hope that it will turn out better for you that way...It won't! You need to take things gradually, whether it's your diet, your workout session, the amount of weight you're lifting, just about everything you do! Keep in mind that any large changes in your lifestyle may even damage your organism, so be realistic and take it easy!

PATIENT EATING IS KEY!

Just as you want to eat less, you'll want to eat less *quickly* now that you're seeking to lose weight. Yes, resting your cutlery while eating and spending more time chewing will do miracles for you, and soon you'll realize you'll be more comfortable eating less or smaller portions because you take the same time you did eating larger ones. Even the simple details are important here!

Don't skip breakfast!

Breakfast has been named "the most important meal of the day" by experts though recent studies have shown it's not always the case. Nevertheless, the benefits of going out with a full stomach cannot be ignored, and having a healthy breakfast at home keeps you from feeling hungry once you're out and buying some fast food. You cannot keep your body from being hungry unless you eat, only delay it. So have that important breakfast at home and you'll be set to go to work or class!

TAKE IT EASY ON WEEKENDS AND DAYS OFF!

Don't throw away all of your progress on a crazy night out or a big family brunch. Remember you're not losing weight part-time; this is a full-time commitment, so stick to it! There are many who will stop exercising once Friday arrives, and change their diet back to fast food and fatty snacks, but you should be one of them. Your effort should be constant, 24/7 and persistent!

SMILE, AND ABOVE ALL, LAUGH!

Laughing is such an excellent activity. It's a way to get rid of stress, we feel better after we do it, it's contagious and guess what...you lose calories when doing so! Yep, studies have discovered that one hour of intense laughter will make you burn up to 120 calories! Maybe you won't be laughing "intensely" for 1 hour anytime soon, but watching a sitcom or comedy film or two will get you dropping calories in *no time!* Try it out, and have some fun losing weight!

STAY POSITIVE AND IGNORE ANY DUMB COMMENTS!

People can be naturally envious of other people's accomplishments, that is normal. Try not to pay attention to any negative comments made to put you down! You're a beautiful person whether or not you accomplish your goals. Many people will comment on your progress before you've even given them a chance to prove them wrong, but if you *do* manage to go all the way and get slimmer like you always wanted, be sure to show them how wrong they were *(gracefully, without being hateful)!* Remember, you're trying, and that's the first and most important step to *anything!!*

REARRANGE YOUR ENVIRONMENT!

Not Feng Shui! What I'm trying to say is that now that you have a weight loss thing going on, try throwing out those things that could make you want to break the diet, like magazines with fast food advertising; cake and cookie recipe books and any chocolate bar packages you may have saved as a souvenir. Also, avoid TV channels that will tempt you, as well as asking someone to change the place where the snacks go, just in case your mind betrays your body one night!

FIND A HOBBY YOU CAN DO AT HOME!

You should look at 'House = Chores' and 'Outside = Exercising'. You can exercise at home, even if you don't have any large weights or treadmills! You can easily find videos online that will give you simple sessions of pushups, sit-ups, and other similar exercises, and you could buy an exercise ball for cheap, which is considered an excellent tool for stretching and exercising on your own. Look for ways to optimize your time, because you won't *always* be able to have time to go out and run, or visit the gym.

FOLLOW A SCHEDULE!

Look, nobody has enough time. *Nobody.* Even someone who is unemployed, or who has enough money to live off for the rest of their lives will find their time limited. Which is why the wisest thing to do is to create a realistic schedule that you can follow daily, or weekly. Include your work shifts, an hour for each meal, an hour's rest and your sleeping hours, then go on from there to the time you'll need to exercise, the time you'll need for the gym or running and so on. It will make you more effective, and you'll take your weight loss process much more seriously than if you hadn't!

LOOK FOR LIKE-MINDED PEOPLE TO SHARE YOUR EXPERIENCES WITH!

Thanks to technology we're now closer than ever, and we can instantly become part of a community online with just a single click! Look for those weight-loss groups, those fitness websites, and weightlifting forums and you'll be set for a quicker and more efficient adventure on the path to getting fitter and slimmer! Don't be afraid to add some posts of your own once you've gotten used to it all, so you can share your own experiences with the world. You never know when a shy boy or girl like you might need a boost!

HATE THAT BELLY? BURN IT DOWN WITH SIT UPS AND A HEALTHY DIET!

While you cannot expect a miraculous disappearance of your belly fat, a progressive practice of sit-ups and a healthy diet will make sure you tone those core muscles and turn that jelly-belly into a six-pack! You must be aware how sexy it looks when men and women have a flat stomach that they can show whenever they want, now it's your turn to have one of your own, as well as receive the health benefits of doing this type of exercise! You can do anywhere between 20 and 100 a day, just make sure to combine them with other important exercises.

DINE HEALTHY, DINE EARLY!

Eating your dinner at night time just isn't efficient for your body or for your weight. To begin with, it will mean you'll have to eat more since you'll be hungrier after having spent so many hours without a meal. This is an indirect way of gaining weight, since although you may not realize it; your body will crave more calories. But it gets worse! Due to the fact that you'll probably eat and then go right to bed, you'll be doing your digestion while lying down, which will lead to flatulence (gas), heartburn, acidity and other uncomfortable pains and problems that will either wake you up or make you have a bad morning. Dine early!

PRIORITIZE ON MAKING YOUR OWN FOOD!

You can buy lots of healthy food at the supermarket or at special stores, but there's nothing like making your own, especially when you want to know what's going into the food. Not only will you ensure you make a meal that's tailor-made for your tastes and calorie intake, but you'll also lose some calories by getting busy in the kitchen! How's that for a weight loss tip?

CLIMB LIKE YOUR LIFE DEPENDS ON IT!

In recent years, it's been discovered that rock-climbing is an incredible activity that will burn a great load of calories. It's demanding on your body and can push you to your limits in terms of strength, endurance and agility; but you'll be burning calories in no time. In fact, the numbers are very impressive: More than 800 calories burned in an hour climbing, and around 600 rappelling. Try indoor climbing if you like to keep it safe and cozy!

REMEMBER JUMPING ROPE AS A KID? NOW DO IT FOR REAL!

As kids, we are not aware of how *good* jumping rope is for our body. It turns out that jumping rope for just *ten* minutes will give you the equal number of calories burned as if you had jogged for *fifteen*! The best part is that you don't even have to leave the square you're standing on to jump rope, and all you need is the rope itself since you could do it barefoot and in pajamas if you're okay with it! Combine it with other indoor exercises and you should be burning plenty of calories without going anywhere.

WAITING ROOMS? MORE LIKE FAT-GAINING ROOMS!

The title of this tip might be a bit cruel, but you have to understand: you can't be sitting around as much as you used to anymore. Avoid waiting rooms, and sitting as you wait for the bus or train. Don't run for a seat on the bus or spend hours on a chair when you're at an office or clinic! You *need* exercise, don't forget. You can stand up, you can walk. Try to take a look around, or at least, stay upright when you're waiting. Also, if it matters to you, people will *notice* that you're avoiding being a lazy bum, and you'll be a positive influence to other people who may also want to start a weight-loss regime.

No More Selective Parking!

I had wanted to get to this one for a while. For those who have worked hard enough to get their own car: it's all well and good to have your means of transport, but be aware that many people will instantly start gaining weight once they do! Having a car eliminates the need to walk to get a bus or train, the need to ride a bicycle or walk at all really since you can park at the very door of the place you're visiting. Try **not** parking so close to places you're visiting. Park far away and *walk*, it's the best way to lose easy calories in a quick manner. Do it for your own health!

UNSURE OF THE BALANCE ON YOUR PLATE? CHECK OUT THE COLORS!

Surprisingly, the number of colors on your plate can indicate how balanced your plate is. Now don't be silly and suggest throwing sprinkles all over your food, what I mean is, add some carrots, broccoli, tomato, lettuce to a (lean, cooked with low-fat oil) steak and a bit of rice or beans and you'll notice how much healthier it will be than a plate with steak, fries and rice. Get what I mean? Colorful salads will always be healthier than dull meats, have that in mind and get your artistic sense flowing when you cook!

MAKE SURE YOU CHOOSE THE RIGHT MEAT TO EAT!

You're allowed to eat meat, we're Omnivores after all (Unless you're vegetarian/vegan, and that's actually better off for weight-loss in the long run, so good for you!). You have to make sure to purchase the right meat, and make sure you cut off the excess fat before cooking it. The best low-fat meats are: Seafood such as Shellfish (Shrimp or crab) or Finfish; Fish such as Salmon or Mackerel; Chicken, Chicken Breast specifically; (Surprisingly) Pork, Tenderloin cuts if possible; Beef Sirloin and Lamb. Organic versions of these products are safer and healthier. Cook them with a soft brush of olive oil for the best results, then enjoy!

JOG AS OFTEN AS YOU CAN!

Despite your efforts at eating well, you simply cannot lose weight without exercise. Make sure you're spending some daily time (1 to 1 1/2 hours) jogging. It doesn't need to be very far from home; just taking a few laps around your block after a good stretch should be enough to get your necessary exercise. Combined with a strict diet, your results will arrive in no time! Diets will save calories, but only exercise and moving around will burn them.

FIND THE FIBER IN YOUR LIFE!

Your body needs fiber if you want to stay healthy *and* lose weight. Fiber brings a long list of benefits to our body, like for example supporting our digestive system and maintaining our immunity. Fiber makes sure your guts (so to speak) are working right, and keeps those good bacteria fed so they can keep doing what they do best. It will also make sure you go to the bathroom like you should, which is a way to avoid *other* issues. The recommended daily intake is 25 to 30 grams, and it can be found in fruits, vegetables, and legumes, but *especially* in whole grains like Cereals, Bread, Flour, Rice and Pasta.

Not a Sporty Person? Try other Fat-burning Activities!

I've already mentioned many options when seeking activities to burn those calories, but most of them have been sports, like swimming, soccer and so on. I talked about Yoga, but maybe that's not your thing either. Well, there's still hope for you! Do you like dancing? Salsa is one excellent way to burn calories. What about stair climbing? Just like a famous boxer did in the movies. Martial Arts and fighting? No? What about riding a bike? There are plenty of options, ***use your imagination!***

So you can't even step outside? You look Great! Come on!

One of the biggest problems for people that prevents them from losing weight isn't a lack of desire, but a lack of self-esteem. We've all been there, the burning desire to go to that gym but without having to face the other guys and girls that go there; the fear of your neighbors watching you jog past their homes; the whispering of those old ladies as they see you in those shorts. Ignore all of that, and *think:* **Who matters more here? ME? Or THEM?** If your answer is the former, then you've got your brain in the right mindset. Now go out and do it without giving a darn!

BE SURE YOU KNOW EXACTLY WHAT YOU WANT!

Many people will just want to lose weight without thinking of the results other than imagining themselves in a sexy bikini or with a powerful chest and abs. You have to *know* what you're gonna work on! Are you going for big, powerful muscles? Do you prefer the final results to be a strong but lean body? Do you want a bigger, fitter butt or legs? Make sure you know what you're aiming for; your exercises will fully depend on it! In fact, even your diet will depend on it!

NO MORE EXCUSES; THIS ISN'T A FAVOR, IT'S A COMMITMENT!

So you have class all morning and then you have to study for tomorrow's exam…**Tough luck!** Every day you'll have to *do* something, nobody lives a life where they can always do what they want! Try to find a way to fit *all* of your commitments into your schedule, and if you can't, something is failing. Perhaps it's your planning, so don't be afraid to admit it and review how you're doing things.

THE EXPERTS KNOW BEST, DON'T BE AFRAID TO ASK!

Personal trainers and Sports instructors exist for a reason. You can always teach yourself something, but the best lessons come from those with experience! If you're at a gym or practicing a sport and you have the chance to learn from somebody who has been doing what you're learning for years, don't be afraid to ask them anything you need. Even if they charge you, it will be much better in the long run since you won't make the mistakes that they made in their beginnings. The student surpasses the teacher in many cases!

DISCOVER YOUR TRUE IDEAL WEIGHT!

Remember: All bodies are different! Maybe for your best friend, weighing a hundred pounds is healthy, but for you, it may be considered *underweight*. Make sure to find out necessary information about what weights and leanness you should be aiming for before you start with a nutritionist or similar expert. Otherwise, you'll have a *new* and *ironic* problem on your hands: Needing to **gain** weight!

No more Oil or Butter: Get a non-stick pan!

Cooking with oil can become an excuse since you'll be tempted to say: "Hey, it's a pain to clean the frying pan if my food's stuck on it!" But if you go out and purchase a non-stick pan, that won't be a problem anymore. If you *must* cook with some oil, give the food a slight brush of olive oil after adding a few spices and enjoy! A healthier option, and in the case of the new pan, an investment!

DON'T PUT YOUR HEALTH AT RISK FOR AN EXTRA DAY OF GYM OR JOGGING!

Just like the title says, if you woke up with a horrible cold, stay at home once you're finished at work. Grab a hot cup of tea and watch some movies. There's a commitment, but it can wait. You're losing weight to stay healthy, so risking your health to lose weight is kind of confusing and silly, right? Also applies if you have a splitting headache or for women in *those* days of the month.

ALSO, DON'T RISK WORSENING AN INJURY FOR A FEW BURNED CALORIES!
Exactly like the above tip. If you feel you pulled a muscle last night during your jog at the beach, or you twisted your ankle when you were going for that ball…Don't force yourself to exercise. Even the best sportsmen get injured, some even career-ending. Think of that whenever you keep exercising after an injury. You're not earning a million-dollar salary and surrounded by the best medical staff, so take it easy now! It could affect other parts of your life.

KIDS KEEPING YOU FROM EXERCISING? NOT IF YOU PLAY WITH THEM!

Ha! I find it funny when people say that since they're parents now, it's all over for them in terms of exercising and losing weight. That's *no* excuse! Your kids are in fact the best fitness companions you could have. They have high energy and they *love* playing around. So go out and kick a ball around, race them and have *fun!* It will help you bond with the wonderful little angels (or devils...just kidding!) and they'll have some great memories of their childhood!

READ-THE-LABELS!

This one is in caps. I have to stress this. Whatever a food package might say on the front, it's the back (or side) — where the nutritional information is — that you should be looking at! There are many 'surprises' that you'll discover in terms of fats, sugars, calories and added preservatives. You need to be aware of what you're eating. After all, your body is a temple like I've said previously. Don't trust any "healthy" foods until you're *sure* that they're healthy. Learn to recognize these things or you'll regret it later!

NOT HELPING MUCH AT HOME? GET INVOLVED!

Many of these tips have talked to the reader as if they're the housewife or the provider of the home, but quite a few reading this book will be sons and daughters, cousins and uncles that are living at their home and taking for granted the effort of others. My suggestion, *get involved* in the work in or around the home! Not only will you burn calories by sweeping, cleaning, taking out the trash, walking the dog or going on errands, you'll also gain the respect and gratitude of those living with you!

ENJOY YOUR VIDEO GAMES? WHY NOT TRY OUT SOME FITNESS ON THEM?

In the last decade or so, technology has taken great leaps, and video gaming hasn't been an exception. Now, you can easily find game titles with features such as cooking, raising pets, baking, creating virtual families and even working out! Many grown-ups use their kid's consoles to work out, and reviews have been greatly positive, with signs of a similar efficiency to having a workout session at a gym! So grab that console, stand on that mat (or other accessory) and get to work. Your kids or younger siblings will laugh their butts off at you, but it's worth it!

SAFETY FIRST: DON'T GO OUT WITHOUT THE RIGHT KIT FOR YOUR WORKOUT!
Whether it's kickboxing or jumping rope, always research what kind of gear you'll need to be using to practice your activities to avoid injuries! Footwear is always the first issue; if you're going running or jogging get some decent shoes with a good sole that can absorb the shocks of running for hours. If you're going to play soccer, get the right fit, with or without studs depending on the surface you'll be on. For basketball there is also a specific type of shoe and so on. As for other gear, light clothing is basically always the go-to kit. Make sure to dress accordingly and use the right gear!

LESS SLEEP, MORE EXERCISE? NO, MORE SLEEP, MORE EXERCISE!

Getting four or five hours of sleep so you can go running in the morning is *not* what you'll want to be doing. A lack of sleep has been proven to work as a complete countermeasure to weight loss. It dulls your mind, and makes you less effective at concentrating yourself and giving more of your effort. It makes you hungrier during the day, so you'll eat more; and finally: You're less likely to drop fat when exercising due to hormonal functions. Get some Z's (7 hours are recommended)!

YOUR BED ISN'T JUST FOR SLEEP THOUGH...*WINK*

Perhaps your partner decided to pass on exercising with you. Still, there's another kind of exercise the two of you can do once you're together in bed...An intense hour of making out can burn 68 calories; having sex for an hour can burn around 150 calories and using your hands or mouth will give you a nice 100 or 200 calories burnt per hour respectively. Bet you didn't know *that!* So get to work, you little devil!

PROTEIN SHAKES AREN'T JUST FOR MUSCLE-HEADS!

I've noticed a misconception from many people who start losing weight. They think that if they drink Whey Protein they'll suddenly become hulking monsters of brawn and muscle. *You won't!* You will however, be replacing weight in fat, for weight in muscle. Benefits will also show in your strength, a reduction in hunger, less probabilities of getting prostate or colon cancer; as well as improving your immune system. Don't seem so bad now do they?

Best time of day for Weight Loss? In the Morning!

Your body's metabolism is in its peak state in the morning, which is why it is recommended by experts to do any exercise sessions in the morning for best results, as well as heavy eating. You'll be burning calories more effectively, and you'll be fresher since you had a good night's sleep after some great sex like I recommended above!

IF IT'S SOMETHING YOU CAN'T LIVE WITH...DON'T LIVE WITHOUT IT!

We've talked all this time about sacrificing, compromising and learning to let go. But there are certain things that are harder to give up than others. If you just can't live without the odd donut, or a bit of cream-cheese or fried foods...Then fine. Keep eating them. We're trying to lead a healthy life here, not a depressing one! But make sure you're controlling your calories elsewhere, so the whole process doesn't fall apart because of one little craving.

BE CAREFUL WITH WHAT YOU'RE TOLD!

I'm not saying every word in this book has to be followed as gospel, but I'd rather you follow my tips and advice than believe what some lady at work told you about mixing some strange herbs into a tea and drinking them. Some people like to give advice without ever confirming if the rumors are true. Avoid drinking, eating or taking any sort of food or medicine without making sure it's good for you! You could end up in the E.R!

ALSO, DON'T BELIEVE IN MIRACLE FAT BURNERS!

Similarly to the previous tip; you'll often see some Miracle Pill on an infomercial that can burn 10 pounds in a week without you going anywhere; or a weird belt that can give you abs if you wear it while watching TV. All of that is simply **B.S (Excuse my French)!** Don't trust those inventions, because if they were *that* good, they would have been announced and sold worldwide, and not on some midday, 20-minute-long infomercial with bad acting. Be realistic!

No pain, No Gain!

I'm not talking about weight-gain. I'm talking about results. You've heard that line before, I'm sure. It's not just something people to say to look hard. If you're exercising, try to push your limits. Don't go out and get injured, but don't give up at your first try. Keep going, run that extra mile, lift the weights an extra time. Check how many calories you're eating and try to eat even *less* without putting your health at risk. The harder you try, the better you'll do, that's a universal law. *Believe in yourself!*

EXHAUSTION IS A GOOD SIGN!

Let me be the first to tell you: If you're exercising and the hour has passed and you feel like you could run for another hour...You're not doing it right! The best trainers will tell you to put as much effort as you can into your workout sessions, and make sure you're training until you're tired. If you're training in the evenings (due to work or class), this will also mean you'll go right home to collapse in your bed. That means more and better sleep in the long term!

IT's a Myth that you need to be rich to Lose Weight!

Some people like to use the excuse that to lose weight you need some extra kind of money to buy healthier food and go to the gym. That's actually not true. As you've noticed by now, I haven't even told you *you have* to go to the gym, or that you *have* to buy a non-stick pan. These are all just tips. You can lose weight simply by doing more chores at home, or jogging around your block with an old, ugly pair of shoes. You can also swap the food you'd normally buy for healthier things, and watch some trainer videos online instead of looking for a trainer in real life. There's actually *no excuse* in this day and age not to start losing weight!

GO OUT, EVEN IF IT'S ALONE!

Like I've been saying for a while now, you don't have to go to the gym, and you don't even have to leave your home to lose weight...But it's always helpful if you go out and have a walk, get off your couch, go partying and dancing. This is more of a motivational tip and less of a weight-loss tip. You'll lose weight, but you'll also enjoy life more than if you're stuck in your home all day! Go out and *do* stuff! You're young and beautiful (I don't care how old you are, reader, the facts are the same)!

HEALTHY COMPETITION IS JUST THAT: HEALTHY!

Starting to workout with somebody else, or beginning a diet at the same time as your best friend is always positive! And as for competing...well that can only go well for the both of you, if you're respectful to each other! Having someone to measure your success against is excellent; since you can make sure you're always doing your best for yourself and for the competition. Just make sure you're not going *too hard on yourself* to win. It's not about winning, it's about losing weight and getting healthy, **don't forget!**

SHOWER INSTEAD OF HAVING A BATH!

It might not be obvious at first, but you can certainly burn more calories by standing around scrubbing and washing the dirt and sweat out of your hair than by lying in a bath and not doing anything much. If you add some dancing in the shower you'll add to the exercise and have a more effective weight-loss hygiene moment every morning. That's certainly a way to kill two birds with a single stone!

Don't kill the Flavor!

Make sure your healthy foods aren't *just* healthy, but also tasty. Find out delicious recipes for your favorite new dishes, otherwise your diet will be nothing but a horrible sacrifice you're doing, and not a yummy new variation to your meals. Think about it: Are you enjoying your diet? If no, then **do something about it!**

THE BEST MOMENT TO EXERCISE MIGHT NOT ACTUALLY BE THE BEST!
That sounds confusing, but what I mean to say is: Despite exercise being better in the morning, if you take a look outside and it's snowed, it's better off if you wait for the afternoon to begin. Similarly for a warm environment, don't worry if you have to wait for sunset to start. Exercising in extreme hot or cold conditions can and will bring excessive shivering or sweating, which can in turn cause fatigue, dizziness and fainting. Be a good judge of the conditions and make a decision!

TIRED OF SALADS? GET SOME SOUP!

Soups are a healthy and tasty option to your diet. They contain less calories than normal food (Since they contain a lot of water — we talked about this previously); possess a large amount of protein and will make you feel as full if not *more* full than when eating a plate of solid food. Try it out, and enjoy! You can turn pretty much *anything* into soup, you'll be surprised!

Reap the Rewards!

You can't always go around chastising yourself for errors if there's no reward for the things you *do* get right! Find a way to treat yourself for reaching a certain milestone; take a day off and have a (low-calorie) treat, go shopping, watch a movie. Perhaps your partner or friends can even become a part of this and reward you for what you've accomplished!

KEEP A RECORD OF WHAT'S GOOD FOR YOU AND WHAT'S NOT!

Not necessarily a journal, but make sure you're aware of what's worked for you and what's not. Perhaps you read on a website that "X food is better than Y", but it simply didn't work out or you didn't like how it tasted. Why is this a good idea? A) Because if you ask an expert about their opinion, you'll need to tell them what you've been eating and doing, and B) You never know when you might end up writing a book or blog about your own experiences losing weight, so you'll need to have a record of everything you did. Sounds good, huh?

Breathe in, Breathe out; Breathing before Eating!

Fitness experts and nutritionists recommend taking ten *deep* breaths after sitting down and before eating a meal. Not only will it help lower levels of built-up stress, but you will speed up your metabolism and achieve an improved digestion and nutrient absorption. Deep breathing is seen as an excellent benefit to your health. Make sure you breathe into your abdomen, not just your chest (shallow breathing) for the best results!

SMALLER PLATES; SMALLER PROBLEMS!

You can always reduce the size of your portion, but how can you be sure if it's enough, or still too much? Well there's an easy option: Get a smaller plate! Since we have the cultural need to avoid wasting food (Which is an excellent view on things) we usually eat everything that we have served before us. A smaller plate means we'll eat a full serving, but in smaller portions than normal. Less calories, while still maintaining a balance.

GOING OUT SOMEWHERE? DON'T EXPECT THE UNKNOWN, EAT AT HOME!

If you're going to a party or meeting, make sure to eat something light and healthy before leaving. Once food starts being served, you'll be tempted to eat, but not if you're already full from eating at home! Do this to avoid having chips, fries, pastries and other greasy foods typically served at social gatherings. Also choose water whenever you can over beer. Wine if you *must* drink alcohol!

THE GOLDEN RULES!

While there are 101 tips to lose weight in this book, the following is a very basic and general one you'll need to memorize. Experts recommend eating three fruit servings a day as well as drinking eight glasses of water. Chicken and Turkey are the best meats to eat (not fried), and make sure to jog at least 30 minutes per day. Drink a glass of cold water after waking up, and don't sit for more than five hours in a row without taking a rest and walking around. There, summed it up for you and everything!

GET YOUR HEART BEATING AND YOUR FAT BURNING WITH CARDIO!

You cannot exercise without cardio, so make sure you're getting those necessary miles of running. But it isn't just about jogging or running. Treadmills do a similar job, as does spin class (great for leg strength and a better butt); jumping rope has a very similar effect to running, like I've said previously; and stair-climbing will strengthen those legs. There are dozens of other ways, ask trainers at the gym or look it up online. You'll love your cardio.

"BUT I WANT TO LOSE WEIGHT, NOT GET STRONGER!" UGH!

Look, all exercise is good for you. I just *hate* when people concentrate on "weight-loss" exercises and don't bother to take the opportunity to improve all around. Why not go for some strength training while you're at it? Some muscle endurance workouts? It's not all about weight-loss, not 100% I mean! And anyway, you'll be burning calories even if you're lifting weights, so don't pass on the chance to develop your muscles! You'll see the difference!

IF YOU CAN'T MANAGE TODAY, YOU WILL TOMORROW, OR AFTER!

Muscle Endurance is increased with gradual increase in repetition. What this means is, if you start by lifting say, 20 pounds, and 30 seems *way* beyond your capacity, then don't lift it! But slowly increase your weight by 2 to 5 pounds, and before long you'll realize how that guy in the corner who can easily lift a hundred pound got to that stage! Endurance is key, and gradual increases with each repetition will guarantee your muscle development.

DON'T THINK OF TAKING BREAKS!

Many people, especially older people, like to take breaks in their weight-loss "periods". Losing weight is a hard enough process on its own for you to go and throw away all the effort — because that's *exactly* what will happen if you go back to your old ways — so don't take your own work for granted and keep going until you've got the desired results!

EAT LIKE YOU'RE POSH!

An effective way to make sure you eat less is by making sure to eat with cutlery (Even if it's pizza or fries), and cutting your food into tiny morsels. You may feel silly, but it definitely guarantees that you'll be full before long! Enjoy your meal and take it slowly!

CHEWING MAKES THE DIFFERENCE!

Our grandma always told us to chew for at least 30 seconds before swallowing. Why? Well at first we thought it was just grandma being grandma, but it turns out that chewing many times before swallowing and taking your time between each bite is an excellent way of feeling full before you actually *are* full. Rest between bites and chew on that food until it's tiny!

DON'T OBSESS; YOUR FUN ADVENTURE COULD TURN INTO A HORROR STORY!

Be careful: Everything in excess is bad for you. Weight-loss should only go *so* far. Once you find the ideal weight, stay there and maintain a healthy lifestyle! Don't keep going and reducing calories or dieting more than you need to. Your body could suffer the consequences, and just how stopping the process could have damaged your hard work, continuing the process beyond the limit will also destroy everything you've worked for. Be wise, don't be hard on yourself!

THE PERFECT DIET!

...Doesn't exist. Don't believe anyone who talks about it. There are tonnes of diets out there, but the one you like most and gives you the best results is the *only* one that matters. Stop thinking that you need to change your diet because so-and-so told you. Only do it if you wish to, and it will help you lose weight *for real.*

PAY GREAT ATTENTION TO THESE TIPS!

These tips have been compiled for you, the reader, after hours of research and many expert opinions. You will need to apply many of them in your near future if you want to guarantee a successful loss of weight, so feel free to regularly look up the most interesting of the tips in this book. And be sure that you *will* achieve results once you're done!

ENJOY EVERY MINUTE!

If you're not having fun with what you're doing...*something is seriously wrong.* Have fun with this entire process and look at it as an **adventure**, because that's what it is. Everything will work out just as you want it, and if you keep a positive attitude and a smile, results will arrive much sooner than you had expected! I wish you all the luck in the world, you beautiful, hard-working person!

BELIEVE IN YOURSELF, ALWAYS!

FINAL NOTES

Hello again!

Well, with all of those excellent tips now in your hands, you should be ready to go out and face the world with a different stance. You are *ready* and the best of all is that you are *willing!* So go out, workout, eat healthy and enjoy.

A great lot of effort and hours were put into the creation of this book, so I hope it works excellently for you now and in the future. Remember that if you ever feel happy with the results, you can always lend, sell or recommend it to somebody else, maybe a loved one or friend! That way, you'll be helping someone out just like somebody might have helped *you* out at one point.

If you really loved it and you wish to help me out, you can leave my book an honest review on Amazon.

Thanks again for downloading **Lose Weight Fast: 101 Ways to Lose up to 10 Pounds in 7 Days,** and **Good Luck!**

www.ingramcontent.com/pod-product-compliance
Lightning Source LLC
Chambersburg PA
CBHW072101280526
45788CB00006B/2357